HoneyBee Books:

Book design, Creator, Author
Melissa L. Perez

Nature Photographer
Breece A. Perry

Product Testing
Breece A. Perry
Linda Guglielmo

Introduction

This booklet is to inspire anyone who is willing to learn how to create, cook and experience new foods that not only heal the body but taste delicious.

These recipes are Medical Medium inspired and were created while on my own personal protocol.

Healing the body with food doesn't mean doing without the foods you love but creating the new to enjoy each day .

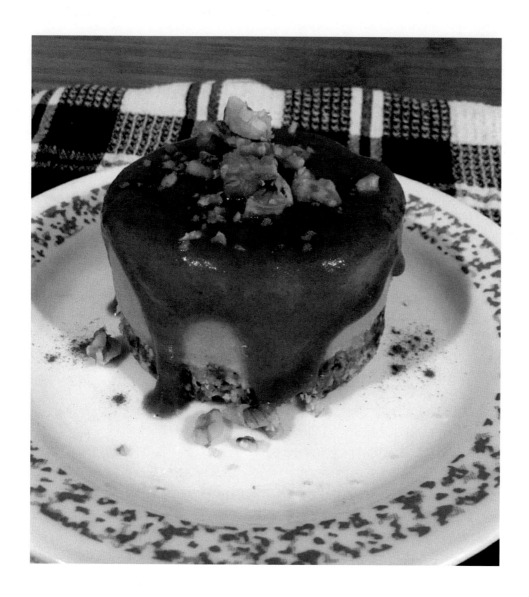

Sweet Surrender Torte

Basic Crumble: (base)
6 dates (pitted, chopped)
1/2 cup almonds
1/4 cup shredded coconut (unsweetened)
1/4 cup raisins
1/4 teaspoon cinnamon

Filling:
1 yam (baked, peeled)
1 teaspoon pumpkin pie spice
1/4 teaspoon cinnamon
3 heaping teaspoons raw wildflower honey
1/3 + 1//4 cups coconut cream
1 tablespoon coconut oil (melted)

Topping:
4 dates (soaked, peeled, pitted)
1 cup coconut cream
1/4 teaspoon pumpkin pie spice
1 tablespoon vanilla
dash of cinnamon
3 teaspoons coconut sugar
walnuts (garnish)

Directions:
For the base crust, blend all the basic crumble ingredients and press into the bottom of three small ramekins or two bigger sized ones. Double the recipe for thicker crust. Spray the ramekins with non-stick coconut baking spray then place either in large baking cups or cut a piece of parchment paper for the bottom of each ramekin which makes it easier to get out when done.

*I used a dark skinned sweet potato or yam
*My choice of raw honey was a local wildflower but you can use any kind you enjoy or even maple syrup would bring an amazing flavor to this dessert.
*I used a potato masher to smash the filling, then into the blender to smooth out. You can use a food processor as well.

Once blended , leave it in the same bowl and make sure it is oven safe. Place into a warm oven for couple minutes only. You will see the mixture melt and becomes nice and smooth. Mix up to make sure it is smooth throughout.

Pour into ramekins covering the base crust and then place into the freezer. Touch the tops checking over a period of 30-45 minutes. When firm , they are set. Then refrigerate until topping is completed.

Blend the coconut cream and dates until smooth as possible then strain. In a small pot on medium to high heat put this mixture along with the rest of the topping ingredients except for the walnuts. Cook it down and watch it closely or it will burn and you will cry! It should become a thick syrup not a paste , rendering about a cup. Pour into a small ramekin and let it cool.

*You do not want to pour this on while hot , it will melt your beautiful masterpiece. Leave at room temperature to cool.

Remove the ready ramekins from the fridge and go around them on the inside edge with a small butter knife to loosen up. Remove the bottom parchment paper and place on a beautiful serving dish of your choice. Pour the sweet topping over and let it ooze down the sides.

Top with a crumble of walnut and serve. Enjoy!

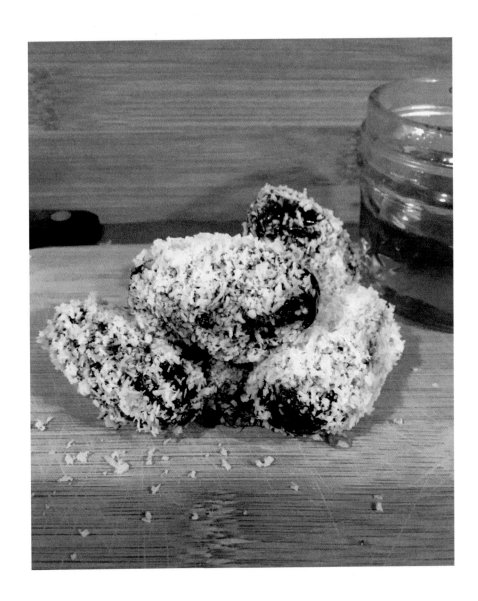

Rolled Dates

Ingredients:
5 dates (frozen)
1 tablespoon Tahini
1 1/2 tablespoons shredded coconut (unsweetened)
3 dashes cinnamon
1 pinch cardamom
1/4 cup raw apple blossom honey

Directions:
Cut the frozen dates down the center and remove the pits.
Mix the tahini and 1 cup of coconut in a small bowl then fill
each date and close it up.
Roll each date in honey and then roll in a mix of the remaining
1/2 coconut and cardamom.

*Dates handle better frozen and keep their shape better when
filling. They should defrost by the time your recipe is
completed.
*If you love pumpkin spice , you can use this in place of the
cinnamon.
*I used apple blossom honey which goes well with the dates
because its so fragrant. Use your favorite honey.

Serve and enjoy!

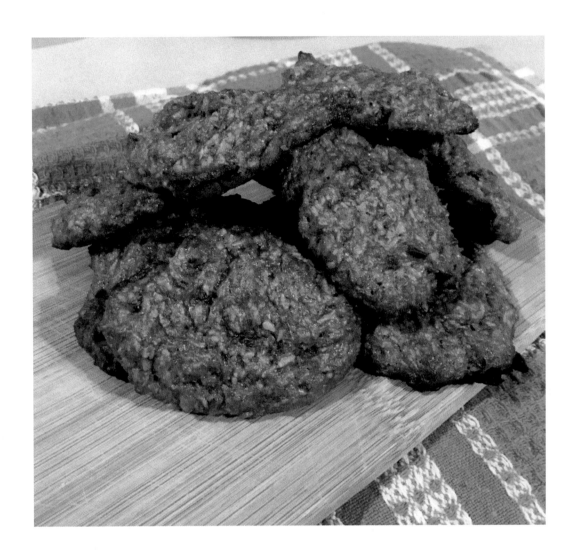

Delish Drop Cookies

Ingredients:
1/3 cup plus 1 tablespoon coconut sugar
1/2 cup organic shredded coconut (unsweetened)
3 tablespoon flax meal
1/4 teaspoon cinnamon
1/3 cup nut butter of choice
1 large plus 1/2 ripe banana (smashed)

Directions:
Mix all dry ingredients then mix all wet ingredients and then mix them both together. Drop onto parchment paper by using a tablespoon . Bake on 350 for 15 to 20 minutes. Take out when the edges are nice and brown.

These cookies are crispy on the outside and soft and chewy on the inside.

*They keep well in the freezer but are so yummy that they are eaten immediately.

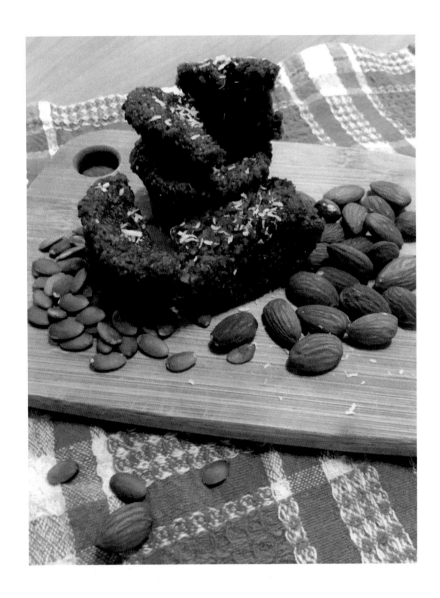

Mimi's Muffins

Ingredients:
2 tablespoons flax meal
6 tablespoons hot water

1 large banana
1 teaspoon vanilla
1/4 cup raw wildflower honey
1 tablespoon molasses
1/2 tablespoon coconut oil
5 tablespoons apple sauce (unsweetened)

1/2 cup almonds
1/2 cup cassava flour
1/4 cup pumpkin seeds
1/4 cup shredded coconut (unsweetened)

1/4 cup raisins
1 teaspoon baking soda
1 1/2 teaspoon baking powder
1/4 teaspoon salt
1/4 teaspoon cinnamon

Directions:
Mix the flax meal and water and let it sit until it thickens
approximately 10-15 minutes.

Mix or blend the second set of ingredients well and set aside.
Blend all of the third set of ingredients until fine then add in the
fourth set of ingredients and mix well. set aside.
Combine all the ingredients in large mixing bowl , mix well.
Fill muffin cups and bake on 350 degrees 20-25 minutes or
until firm to the touch on top and brown. Let cool completely
and put in the fridge.

*They firm up once they have been refrigerated for few hours.
These are very moist and tender muffins.

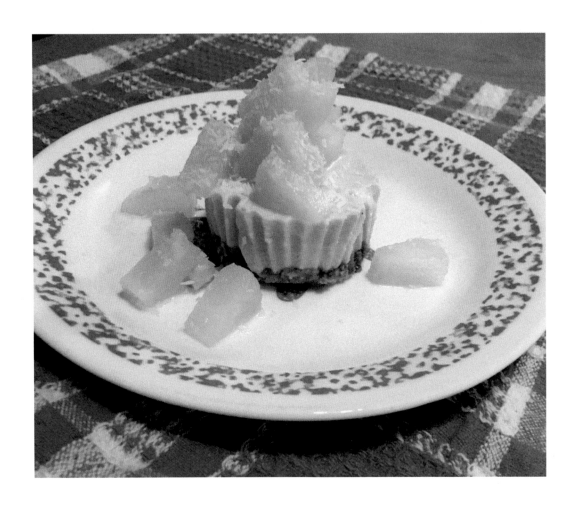

Creamy Coconut Cashew Cups

Crust:
1/2 cup raw almonds
1/2 cup shredded coconut (unsweetened)
1/2 gluten free oats
1/8 teaspoon cinnamon
2 tablespoons raw wildflower honey
pinch of salt
cupcake cups

Filling:
1/2 cup raw cashews (soaked, drained)
1 cup coconut cream
1/4 cup coconut water (see notes)
1/2 teaspoon vanilla
1/4 cup of raw wildflower honey

Topping & Garnish:
2 cups pineapple canned or fresh
2 tablespoons shredded coconut (unsweetened)

Directions:
Blend all crust ingredients well except for the honey. After blended fine then add in honey and mix well. Scoop some into each cupcake cups and press down firm.
Blend all filling ingredients until syrup like or becomes a liquid. You want it super smooth like milk consistency. Pour into the cups and put in the freezer for couple hours to set.

*Soaking the cashews makes the cream smoother.Let it sit about 10 minutes or so or until softened.
*They can be left in the freezer and taken out as needed.
*You can use any fruit you want as topping. I used canned organic coconut milk.
*I leave in the fridge over night so the cream settles on top that yields a cup. Left is the remaining coconut water to take from for the 1/4 cup needed.

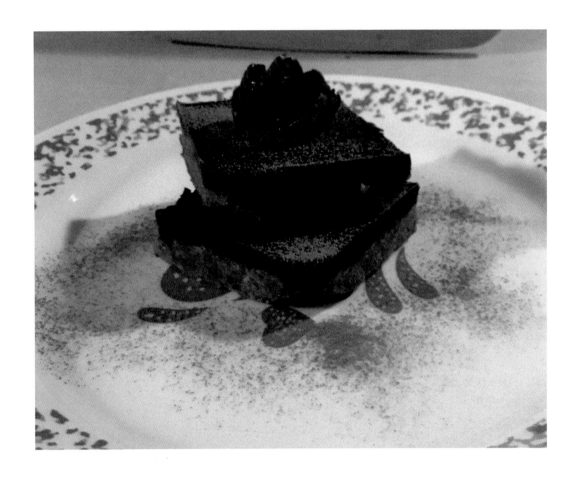

Date Nut Bar With Dark Chocolate

Ingredients:
1 cup extra dark chocolate chips 85% (mini's)
1/2 tablespoon coconut oil

Basic Crumble:
6 dates (pitted, chopped)
1/2 cup raw almonds
1/4 cup shredded coconut (unsweetened)
1/4 cup raisins
1/4 teaspoon cinnamon

Directions:
Blend all of the basic crumble ingredients until the mixture comes together. Press the crumble down into a 6x6 sandwich container using a measuring cup to flatten smooth. Make sure to spray it first with some coconut oil non stick baking spray. (container substitute: use four -X large parchment baking cups)

Bring a small pot of water to a boil then take off the heat and set aside. Put the oil and the chocolate chips into a metal bowl and place over top of the pot and let it sit for a few minutes then stir until the chocolate and oil are melted together. Pour on top of the crust base. Place in the freezer until it hardens.

Serve with chopped dates on top and a dash of cinnamon.

*Sunflower seeds , walnuts or hazelnuts can also be used as a nut for the basic crumble and would add amazing flavor!

*Mini chocolate chips melt faster.

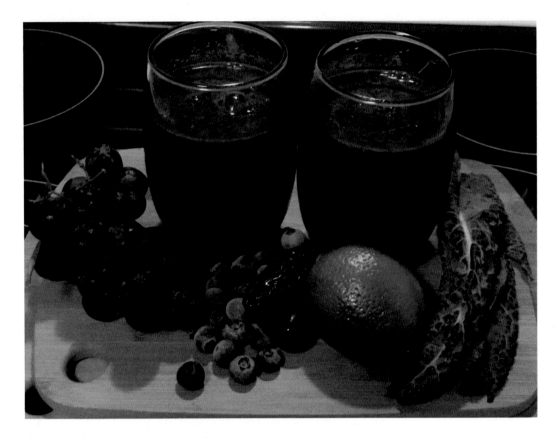

Breakfast Smoothie

Ingredients:
juice of 1 lime
handful kale
bunch black grapes
2 dates (pitted)
handful blueberries
1 cup organic black cherry juice

Directions:
Blend all and serve in your favorite glass.

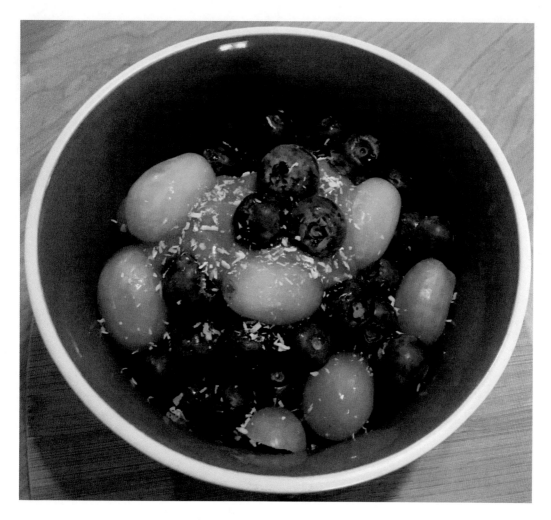

Breakfast Bowl

Ingredients:
1/2 cup green grapes
1/2 cup blueberries

Topping:
shredded coconut (unsweetened)
1 teaspoon tahini
1 tablespoon creamed raw honey
dash cinnamon

Directions:
In a mixing bowl add tahini, honey and cinnamon and stir. Put a dollop of topping over the fruit and sprinkle with coconut.

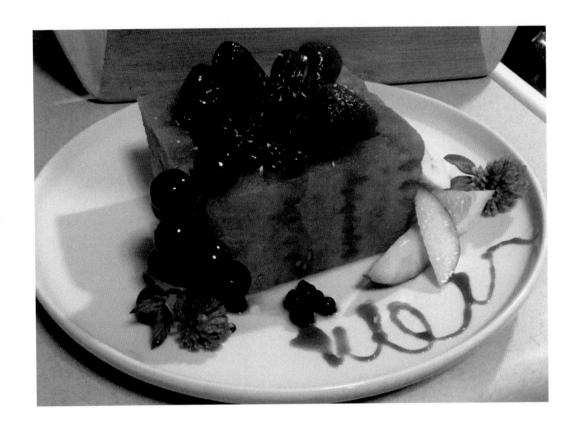

Watermelon & Fruit Art

1 small sweet watermelon
few black grapes (left on the vine)
2 dates
3 strawberries
couple nectarine wedges
small slice banana
1 lemon wedge
few wild blueberries
few black cherries
couple red clover flowers
raw clover honey (drizzle)

I cut off the bottom of the watermelon so it sits flat. Then the sides and top to form a square. I cut a smaller square into the top leaving 1/2" for the rim of the bowl then sliced downward on each side careful not to slice through to the bottom. I used a melon baller to scoop out the center of the square creating the space/bowl.
Once completed, I placed some of the blueberries and cherries in the bottom to take up room creating a platform. I then placed more up toward the surface of one side, then the strawberries and then the dates right on top . I anchored a grape in the corner under a few blueberries and draped it down over the side corner and on to the plate surface. I then placed a red clover flower there. I scattered a few blueberries in front then on the other side. I placed a couple peach wedges, a lemon wedge and a sliced piece of banana and next to that another red clover flower. I drizzled a swirly design across the front of the plate using the clover honey.

*With a small art brush I brushed honey over the fruit in the basket for shine.
*Its fun to practice knife skills on a larger watermelon that allows for two square bowls rather than one.

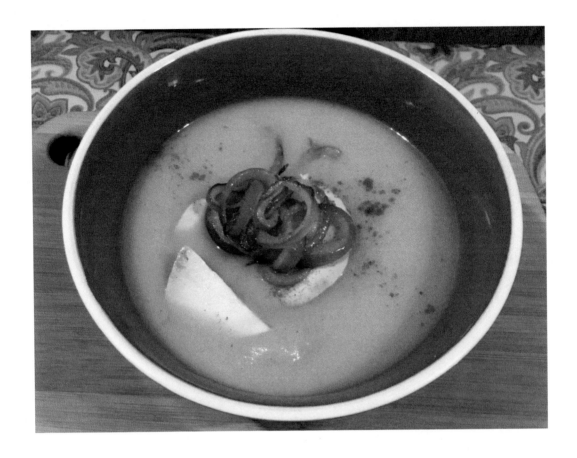

Sweet Potato Soup With Avocado & Curried Onions

Soup:
2 small sweet potatoes
2 cups water (reserve 1/2)
1/2 tablespoon coconut cream (unsweetened)
4 pinches pink salt
1 pinch black pepper
1/8 teaspoon smoked paprika
1/4 teaspoon curry powder

Topping:
1/2 red onion (sliced thin)
1 teaspoon coconut oil
2 pinches curry powder
2 pinches pink salt
1/2 avocado (sliced thick)
dash smoked paprika

Directions:
Roast two small sweet potatoes in the oven on 375 degrees for about 45 minutes to an hour. Use a fork to check for doneness. You should be able to poke a fork through like with ease. when done set aside and let it cool enough to peel. After peeled put into a blender adding the water 1 1/2 cups blend smooth and if still too thick , add the remaining 1/2 cup reserved. It should be thick enough to hold up the avocado slices yet soupy enough to stir easily. To warm, transfer into a small pot.
Add in coconut cream and the spices and stir well until warmed.
Stay with it and make sure to heat it through ,then transfer into your favorite bowl.

In a small sauce pan sauté the onions in the coconut oil and salt for just a few minutes let them caramelize then add in the curry powder , mix, remove from heat and set aside. Top the bowl of soup with the sliced avocado and then curried onions and sprinkle of the smoked paprika.

*You want to balance the sweetness of the sweet potato with the salt . Salt and pepper always to taste and this goes for any spices , if you like more add more if you prefer less then taste first before adding more.
*Also if doing low fat or no fat you can add a teaspoon of coconut cream to the soup instead of tablespoon and can sauté the onions in broth instead of oil.

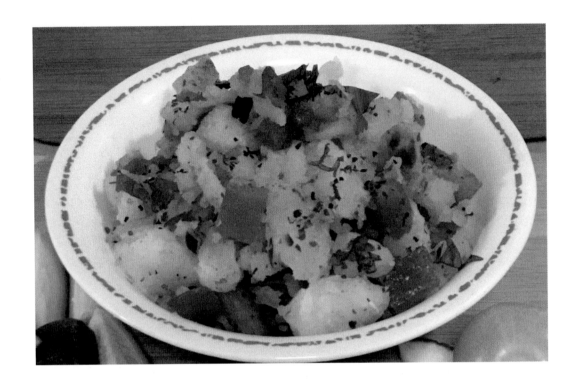

Italiano Potato Salad

Ingredients:
2 large potatoes
4 Rome tomatoes (seeded, diced)
1tiny red onion (diced)
2 basil leaves (chopped)
1/2 teaspoon dulse flakes
1 teaspoon onion powder
1 teaspoon garlic powder
2 tablespoons olive oil
salt & pepper to taste

Directions:
Roast the potatoes in the oven on 375 degrees until fork tender. Let them cool. Peel the potatoes and rough chop them and place them in a medium mixing bowl.

In a small mixing bowl, add the rest of the ingredients and mix well. Dulse flakes are salty so make sure to taste before adding more salt.

*I used cilantro the day I made this recipe, however I change it up depending on what herbs I have on hand. Basil is ideal for this recipe and very aromatic.
*This dish can be eaten warm or cold.

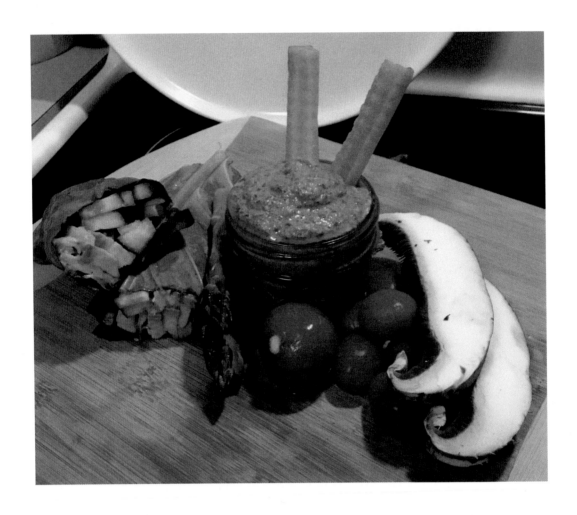

Veggie Board With Dip

Wraps:
1 large collard green leaf
1/2 cucumber
2 large radishes
2 asparagus spears
1/2 avocado

*Slice cucumber, avocado, and radishes long ways. Roll them and the asparagus up in the collard green leaf.
*Place other veggies on the side such as carrots, grape tomatoes, mushrooms and extra radish or asparagus.

Dip:
2 cups cilantro
1 tsp pumpkin seeds
juice 1/2 lemon
1tsp extra virgin olive oil
1 slice jalepeno pepper
1scallion
1/2 garlic clove
2 broccoli (bite size florets)
salt & pepper to taste
1/2 avocado

*Blend all and serve in a small ball jar or bowl.

Dressing used for dipping, drizzling or roasting:

Ingredients:
1 large clove garlic
1/2 teaspoon onion powder
1/8 teaspoon salt
1 tablespoon dulse flakes
1/8 teaspoon smoked paprika
1 tablespoon extra virgin olive oil

Directions:
Put all ingredients into a small mixing bowl and whisk until combined.

*Dulse flakes are salty. Taste first before adding the salt if your diet is salt free.
*This sauce is awesome for roasting potatoes, dressing a raw salad and dipping your veggies or fries in.
*The oil can be omitted in the dip for no fat however, it is needed in the dipping, drizzling and roasting sauce.

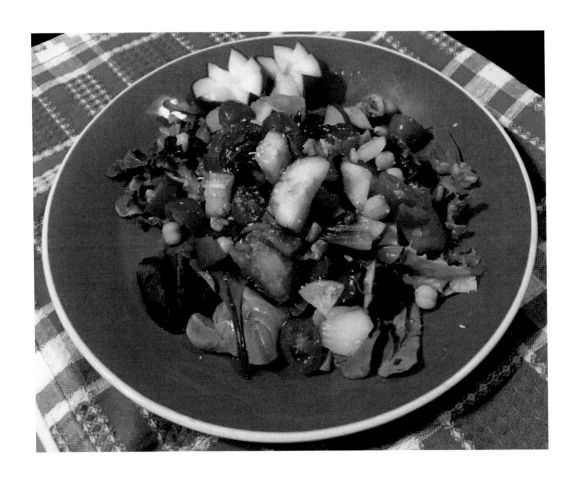

Mega Salad With Spicy Asian Dressing

Ingredients:
2 cups mixed greens
1 cup spinach
2 sweet mini red peppers
1 tiny red onion (diced)
1 mini cucumber (sliced)
1/4 cup raw walnuts (chopped)
1/2 cup grape tomatoes (halved)
2 red radishes (sliced thin)
1/4 cup chick peas
1 ripe apricot (chopped)

Dressing:
1/4 cup liquid coconut aminos
2 tablespoon honey
2 tablespoons lemon juice
1 garlic clove (pressed)
1/2 teaspoon fresh ginger juice
1/2 tsp sesame oil
salt & pepper to taste

Directions:
In a large salad bowl toss all the ingredients together.
In a small mixing bowl whisk all dressing ingredients together
and drizzle over top.

*I used a handheld stainless steel garlic press.

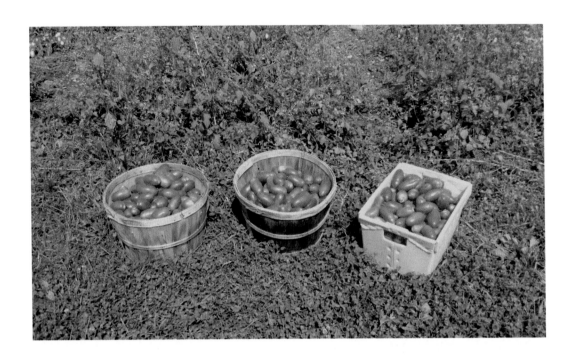

ORGANIC PLUM TOMATOES FROM THE GARDEN

Pomodoro & Garlic Salad

Ingredients:
6 Plum tomatoes (diced)
3 tablespoons extra virgin olive oil
2 garlic cloves (pressed)
2 mini seedless cucumbers (sliced)
1 large portobello mushroom (chopped)
1 teaspoon fresh basil (chopped)
1/2 teaspoon Italian seasoning
1/2 teaspoon onion powder
dash salt & pepper

Directions:
Saute' the diced mushroom until fork tender in 1 tablespoon of the olive oil.
In a large bowl mix all ingredients together.
Best served cold.

Red Lentil Pasta With Eggplant

Ingredients:
1/2 box Red Lentil pasta (linguini)
1 celery stalk (chopped)
1 cup eggplant (chopped)
2 large tomatoes (diced)
1 garlic clove (diced)
1 teaspoon extra virgin olive oil
1/2 teaspoon Italian seasoning
dash black pepper
sprinkle dulse flakes

Directions:
In large pot boil the pasta till done and set aside.
In a sauce pan on medium heat, sauté the celery and garlic
with olive oil first, once translucent add in tomatoes, eggplant
and Italian seasoning. Set on low and let simmer until fork
tender.
Add in the pasta, toss and plate.

*Sprinkle on as much dulse flakes as you would like, I used it
for salt in this dish. Pepper to taste.

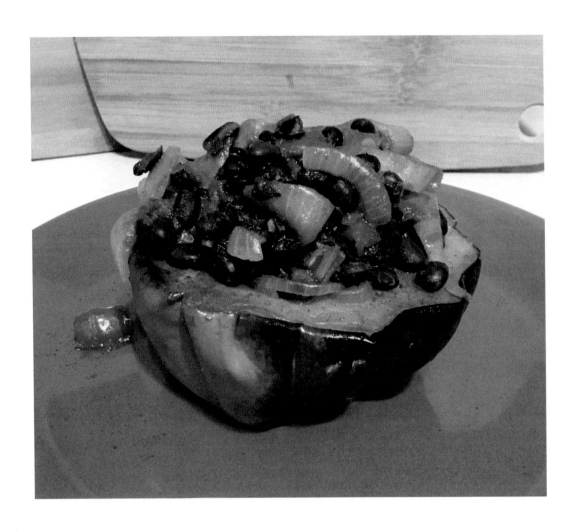

Roasted Acorn Squash With Black Beans

Ingredients:
1 acorn squash
1 can black beans (rinse, drain)
1/2 cup green pepper (diced)
1 medium onion sliced round (pull rings apart)
1/2 cup cilantro (chopped)
1 Plum tomato (diced)
1 large garlic clove (minced)
1 teaspoon olive oil
1/4 cup water
3 pinches salt
1/2 teaspoon garlic powder
1/2 teaspoon onion powder
1/4 teaspoon smoked paprika
1 1/2 teaspoons fresh lemon juice (or Spanish green olives)

Directions:
Split in half and deseed acorn squash. Roast it open faced down. Rub a little olive oil on it first which helps with browning and prevents sticking.
Roast on 375 degrees for about 30-40 min or until fork tender. Remove from oven and set aside.
In medium pot, sauté the onion and peppers in the olive oil until browned. Stir continuously. Add in the salt to sweat the onions and when browned add the tomatoes, beans and cilantro. I used blended, frozen cilantro that is more of a liquid than a solid. If you need more of the 1/4 c water then add more but make sure to keep a thicker consistency. You don't want soup. Add in seasonings, garlic and lemon juice and stir.

*I used lemon juice in place of Spanish olives. If you use olives they also give a wonderful flavor and acidity to this dish. Let it simmer on low heat for about 10 minutes or until the flavors marry. On your favorite plate, place the squash and fill with a generous amount of black bean filling. Sprinkle a little smoked paprika on top.

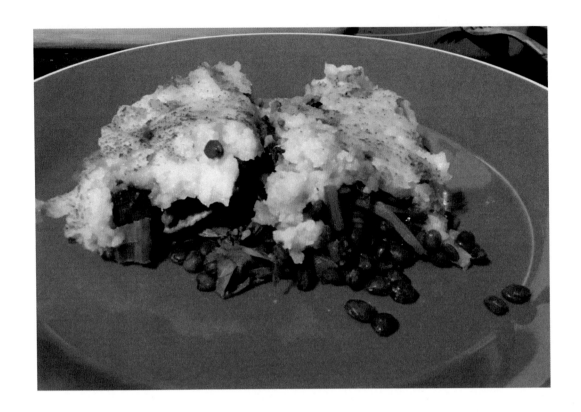

Shepherd's Pie

Filling:
8 ounce package portobello mushrooms (rough chop)
1 can lentils (rinse, drain)
2 celery stalks with leaves (chopped)
2 carrots (chopped)
1/2 teaspoon onion powder
1/2 teaspoon garlic powder
1/4 teaspoon smoked paprika
1 teaspoon Italian seasoning
1 cup peas (defrosted, drained)
salt & pepper to taste

Potato Mash:
5-6 large potatoes (peeled)
1 garlic clove (mashed)
2 tablespoons olive oil
1 dash onion powder
1 dash garlic powder

Directions:
In a baking dish that has a top, put all the filling ingredients and mix and level it out. Mash all potato ingredients together till creamy or bit chunky, however you prefer them but creamy enough to spread. Spread the mash over the filling, cover and bake on 350 degrees. When you see it bubbling on the sides, uncover it and let it brown on top. It should make its own gravy from the mushrooms and veggies. Enjoy!

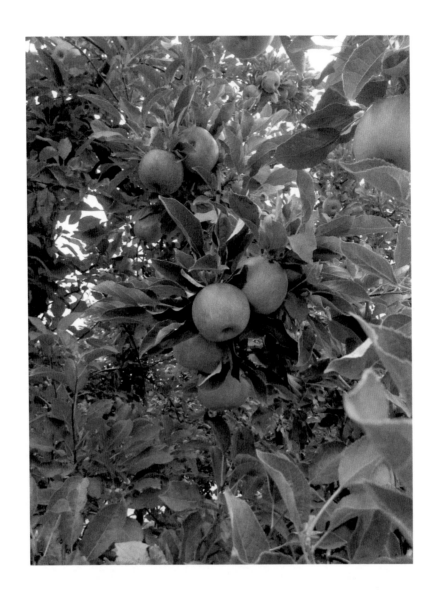

HONEY CRISP APPLES RIGHT FROM THE TREE.

Ribboned Carrot Apple Slaw

Ingredients:
1 carrot (ribboned)
1 Honey Crisp apple (sliced)
2 tablespoons raisins
1/2 teaspoon fresh ginger juice

Topping:
1 tablespoon Tahini
2 tablespoons raw clover honey
1/2 teaspoon shredded coconut (unsweetened)
dash cinnamon

Directions:
In a medium size bowl put all the ingredients and toss.
Combine the tahini and honey then drizzle over the top.
Sprinkle on the coconut and raisins.

*If you leave this for about 20-30 minutes the carrot ribbons
will soften and become easier to chew and digest.
*You can add walnuts or pine nuts to add depth of flavor to this
dish.
*I found this not only filling but refreshing using a Honey Crisp
apple.

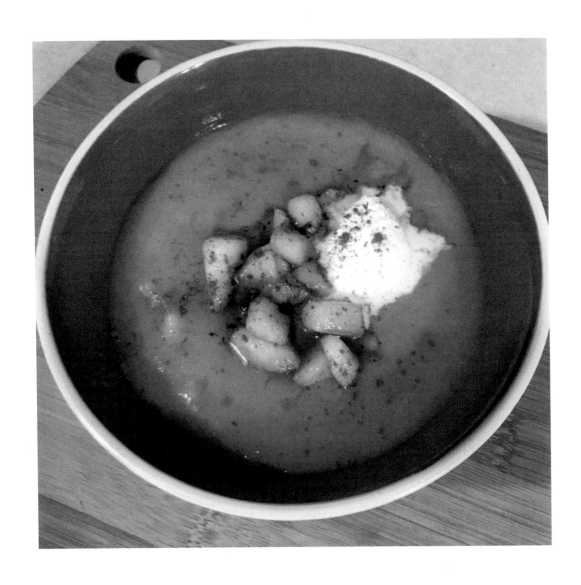

Sinful Apple Millet Porridge

Porridge:
1 small Gala apple (peeled, chopped)
1 Ginger Gold apple (peeled, chopped)
1/2 cup coconut milk
1cup water (reserve 1/2 cup)
1/2 tablespoon vanilla
1/4 teaspoon cinnamon
1 pinch pink salt
2 tablespoons millet flour
1/4 cup pure maple syrup
1 tablespoon potato starch

Topping:
1/2 large tart apple (peeled, diced)
1 tablespoon pure maple syrup
1 teaspoon coconut oil
1 tablespoon coconut cream
2 pinches cinnamon

Directions:
In a blender pulse the two small chopped apples with 1/2 cup of water and 1/2 cup of coconut milk to an oatmeal consistency. (a little lumpy yet blended smooth). Transfer to a medium pot. Add vanilla, salt and cinnamon. Stir on medium heat. Combine the Millet flour with the reserve 1/2 cup of water and stir until dissolved completely (no lumps) and add this in the pot while stirring. After a few minutes spoon out 4 spoonfuls of the cooking mixture into a small cup or bowl and add in the potato starch, stir this quickly until dissolved then pour it back into the pot. Stir and turn up the heat slightly to thicken. Keep stirring and watch it so it doesn't burn. In few minutes it will thicken and bubbles will form coming up through the porridge.

*It should be thick enough to stick to the back of a spoon and roll off slowly like oatmeal would, not runny.

If all looks good, remove from the heat and set aside. Add the maple syrup and stir. Let it sit. As it does i will thicken more.

In a small sauce pan on medium heat add the coconut oil, roll it around the pan to coat it then throw in the tart diced apple. you want to brown it and soften it a bit. Once there, add in the pinch of cinnamon and toss it around in the apples. Let the heat bring out the flavor in the spice then add in the tablespoon of maple syrup and stir well. It will bubble like a glorious symphony! Remove from the heat and set aside.

Pour the porridge into your favorite bowl and top with the scrumptious apples. Top that with the coconut cream and 2 pinches of cinnamon for the final touch!

*Do not add the Millet flour directly into the hot porridge to short cut without stirring into the water first, it will clump up like eggs.

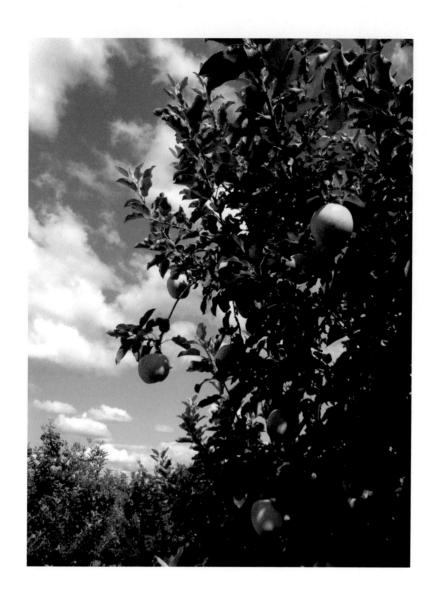

GINGER GOLD APPLES

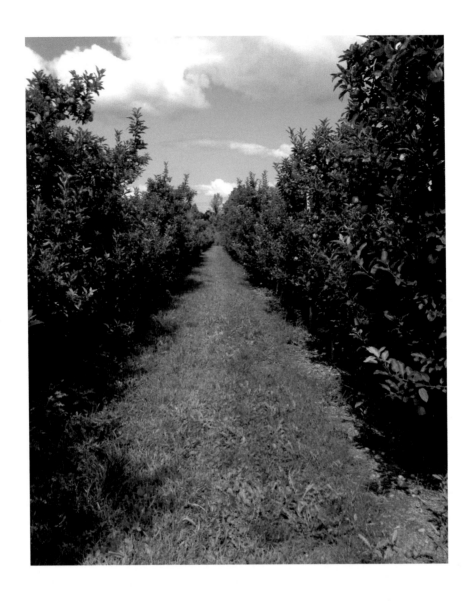

Wether under our feet, above our heads or right in front of our eyes, nature gives us what we need to heal.

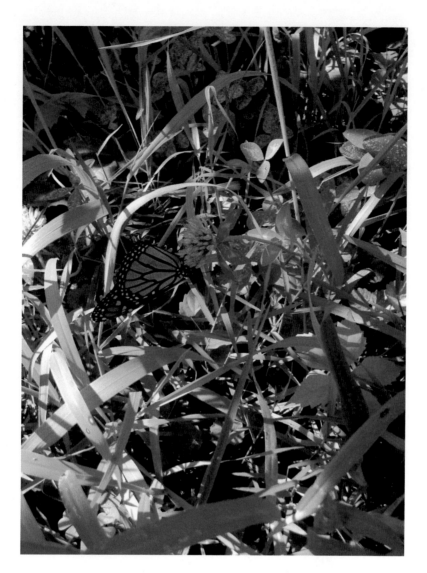

MONARCH ON RED CLOVER

GENERAL INDEX

Introduction, 1-2

Sweet Surrender Torte, 3-5

Rolled Dates, 6-7

Delish Drop Cookies, 8-9

Mimi's Muffins, 10-11

Creamy Coconut Cashew Cups, 12-13

Date Nut Bar With Dark Chocolate, 14-15

Breakfast Smoothie, 16

Breakfast Bowl, 17

Watermelon & Fruit Art, 18-19

Sweet Potato Soup With Avocado & Curried Onions, 20-21

Italiano Potato Salad, 22-23

Veggie Board With Dip, 24-25

Dressing used for dipping, drizzling or roasting, 25

Mega Salad With Spicy Asian Dressing, 26-27

Garden Photo, 28

Pomodoro & Garlic Salad, 28

Red Lentil Pasta With Eggplant, 29

Roasted Acorn Squash With Black Beans, 30-31

Shepherd's Pie, 32-33

Orchard Photo (Honey Crisp Apples), 34

Ribboned Carrot Apple Slaw, 35

Sinful Apple Millet Porridge 36-38

Orchard Photo (Ginger Gold Apples), 39

Conclusion: Orchard Photo (Author Afterthoughts), 40

Orchard Photo (Monarch On Red Clover), 41

Made in the
USA
Middletown, DE